Antoinette Kleinhans

Managing Stress

Breathe, Relax, Succeed: Managing Workplace Stress with Mindfulness

Chapter 1: Understanding Workplace Stress

The Impact of Workplace Stress on Employee Health

Workplace stress is a common issue that affects employees across various industries. The impact of workplace stress on employee health cannot be underestimated. Stress can manifest in various ways, including physical symptoms such as headaches, muscle tension, and fatigue. It can also lead to mental health issues such as anxiety and depression. When left unchecked, workplace stress can have a detrimental effect on employee well-being and productivity.

One of the key ways in which workplace stress affects employee health is through the release of stress hormones such as cortisol. Prolonged exposure to these hormones can weaken the immune system, making employees more susceptible to illnesses. Chronic stress can also lead to cardiovascular problems, digestive issues, and other serious health conditions. Employers need to be aware of the impact of workplace stress on employee health and take steps to mitigate its effects.

In addition to physical health, workplace stress can also have a significant impact on mental health. Employees who are constantly under pressure and feeling overwhelmed are more likely to experience symptoms of anxiety and depression. This can lead to decreased motivation, poor job performance, and even burnout. Employers must recognize the signs of stress in their employees and provide the necessary support and resources to help them manage their stress effectively.

It is essential for employers to create a work environment that promotes employee well-being and reduces workplace stress. This can include implementing stress management programs, providing access to mental health resources, and fostering a culture of open communication and support. By addressing workplace stress proactively, employers can help improve employee health, morale, and overall productivity.

In conclusion, the impact of workplace stress on employee health is significant and cannot be ignored. Employers must prioritize the well-being of their employees by implementing strategies to reduce stress and create a positive work environment. By taking action to address workplace stress, employers can help improve employee health and create a more productive and engaged workforce.

Common Causes of Workplace Stress

Workplace stress is a common issue that many employees face on a daily basis. There are several common causes of workplace stress that can contribute to feelings of overwhelm, burnout, and anxiety. One of the main causes of workplace stress is heavy workloads and staff shortage. When employees are constantly under pressure to complete tasks quickly and efficiently, it can lead to feelings of stress and pressure.

Another common cause of workplace stress is poor communication. When there is a lack of clear communication between managers and employees, it can lead to misunderstandings, conflicts, and increased stress levels. Additionally, a toxic work environment can also be a major contributor to workplace stress. When employees are surrounded by negativity, gossip, and interpersonal conflicts, it can take a toll on their mental health and well-being.

Lack of work-life balance is another common cause of workplace stress. When employees are expected to work long hours, take on additional responsibilities, and constantly be available to work outside of regular business hours, it can lead to feelings of burnout and exhaustion. Finally, a lack of support from management can also contribute to workplace stress. When employees feel unsupported, unappreciated, or undervalued by their managers, it can lead to feelings of frustration, resentment, and stress.

In order to effectively manage workplace stress, it is important for both employees and employers to address these common causes head-on. By promoting open communication, fostering a positive work environment, encouraging work-life balance, and providing support and recognition to employees, workplaces can create a more harmonious and stress-free atmosphere. By understanding the common causes of workplace stress and taking proactive steps to address them, employees can better manage their stress levels and improve their overall well-being in the workplace.

Recognizing the Signs of Workplace Stress

Recognizing the signs of workplace stress is crucial in order to address and manage it effectively. Stress at work can manifest in various ways, both physically and mentally. One common sign of workplace stress is feeling constantly overwhelmed or unable to cope with the demands of your job. This can lead to feelings of anxiety, irritability, and difficulty concentrating on tasks.

Another key indicator of workplace stress is experiencing physical symptoms such as headaches, muscle tension, or stomach issues. These physical symptoms can be a result of the body's response to stress, including the release of cortisol and adrenaline. It's important to pay attention to these signs and take action to reduce stress in order to prevent further health problems down the line.

Changes in behavior can also be a sign of workplace stress. This may include withdrawing from social interactions, increased use of substances like alcohol or tobacco, or changes in eating habits. Recognizing these behavioral changes in yourself or your colleagues can help identify when stress levels are becoming unmanageable and when intervention is necessary.

Emotional signs of workplace stress can include feelings of frustration, anger, or sadness. These emotions may be a result of feeling overwhelmed, undervalued, or unsupported in the workplace. It's important to address these emotional signs of stress in order to prevent burnout and maintain overall well-being.

By recognizing the signs of workplace stress early on, individuals can take steps to manage their stress levels and prevent it from escalating. This may include practicing mindfulness techniques, seeking support from colleagues or a professional counselor, or making changes to work habits and environments. It's important for employers to create a supportive work culture that values employee well-being and provides resources for managing stress effectively. By being proactive in recognizing and addressing workplace stress, individuals can improve their overall health and productivity in the long run.

Chapter 2: Introduction to Mindfulness

What is Mindfulness?

Mindfulness is a practice that involves being fully present in the moment, without judgment or distraction. It is about paying attention to our thoughts, feelings, and sensations with awareness and acceptance. In the context of the workplace, mindfulness can be a powerful tool for managing stress and improving overall well-being. By cultivating mindfulness, individuals can learn to respond to challenges with greater clarity, resilience, and compassion.

One key aspect of mindfulness is focusing on the present moment. This means letting go of worries about the past or future, and instead, bringing our attention to what is happening right now. By staying present, we can better appreciate our experiences and respond to them in a more effective way. In the workplace, this can help us stay focused on tasks, make better decisions, and communicate more effectively with colleagues.

Another important aspect of mindfulness is cultivating awareness of our thoughts and emotions. By becoming more attuned to our inner experiences, we can gain insight into how we are feeling and why. This self-awareness can help us identify patterns of stress or negative thinking, and develop strategies for managing them more effectively. By recognizing our emotions and thoughts without judgment, we can learn to respond to them in a more constructive way.

Practicing mindfulness can also help us develop greater emotional resilience. By staying present and aware of our thoughts and feelings, we can learn to respond to challenges with greater equanimity and compassion. This can help us navigate workplace stress more effectively, and build stronger relationships with colleagues. By cultivating mindfulness, we can develop a greater sense of overall well-being and resilience in the face of workplace challenges.

In summary, mindfulness is a powerful tool for managing workplace stress and improving overall well-being. By practicing mindfulness, individuals can learn to stay present in the moment, cultivate awareness of their thoughts and emotions, and develop greater emotional resilience. By incorporating mindfulness into their daily routine, individuals can create a more balanced, focused, and compassionate approach to work and life.

Benefits of Practicing Mindfulness in the Workplace

In today's fast-paced work environment, stress has become a common issue for many employees. The constant pressure to meet deadlines, handle difficult tasks, and navigate work politics can take a toll on one's mental and physical well-being. However, there is a solution that can help alleviate workplace stress and improve overall productivity - mindfulness. Practicing mindfulness in the workplace has been proven to have numerous benefits that can positively impact both employees and organizations.

One of the main benefits of practicing mindfulness in the workplace is stress reduction. By being fully present and aware of your thoughts, feelings, and surroundings, you can better manage stress and prevent it from escalating. Mindfulness techniques such as deep breathing, meditation, and body scans can help calm the mind and body, leading to a more relaxed and focused state of being. This can result in improved decision-making, better problem-solving abilities, and increased resilience in the face of challenges.

In addition to stress reduction, mindfulness can also enhance interpersonal relationships in the workplace. By practicing active listening, empathy, and compassion, employees can improve communication with their colleagues, managers, and clients. This can lead to better teamwork, conflict resolution, and overall job satisfaction. When employees feel heard, understood, and valued, they are more likely to be engaged and motivated in their work.

Furthermore, mindfulness can boost creativity and innovation in the workplace. By quieting the mind and cultivating a sense of curiosity and openness, employees can tap into their creative potential and think outside the box. This can lead to new ideas, solutions, and opportunities for growth and success. When employees are encouraged to explore different perspectives and approaches, they can contribute to a culture of innovation that benefits the entire organization.

Overall, the benefits of practicing mindfulness in the workplace are numerous and far-reaching. From stress reduction to improved communication, creativity, and innovation, mindfulness can have a profound impact on both individuals and organizations. By incorporating mindfulness techniques into your daily routine, you can create a more peaceful, productive, and harmonious work environment that supports the well-being and success of all employees.

How Mindfulness Can Help Manage Workplace Stress

In today's fast-paced work environment, stress is a common occurrence for many employees. From tight deadlines to demanding bosses, the pressures of the workplace can take a toll on both our physical and mental well-being. However, there is a solution that can help manage workplace stress effectively: mindfulness.

Mindfulness is the practice of being present in the moment and fully aware of your thoughts, feelings, and surroundings. By incorporating mindfulness techniques into your daily routine, you can learn to manage stress more effectively and improve your overall well-being. We will then explore how mindfulness can help you cope with workplace stress and provide you with practical tips on how to incorporate mindfulness into your workday.

One of the key benefits of mindfulness is its ability to help you stay focused and present in the moment. When you are mindful, you are better able to handle stressful situations with clarity and composure. By staying present in the moment, you can avoid getting caught up in negative thoughts or emotions that can exacerbate stress. This can help you make better decisions and respond to challenges in a more effective way.

Mindfulness can also help you cultivate a sense of calm and relaxation in the midst of a hectic workday. By practicing mindfulness techniques such as deep breathing or meditation, you can reduce the physical symptoms of stress, such as tension in the body and rapid heartbeat. This can help you feel more centered and grounded, even in the face of challenging situations at work.

In addition to reducing stress, mindfulness can also help you improve your overall well-being and job performance. By practicing mindfulness regularly, you can enhance your focus, creativity, and problem-solving skills. This can help you become more productive and efficient at work, leading to greater job satisfaction and success.

Overall, incorporating mindfulness into your daily routine can help you manage workplace stress more effectively and improve your overall well-being. By staying present in the moment, cultivating a sense of calm, and enhancing your job performance, you can navigate the challenges of the workplace with greater ease and resilience. So take a deep breath, relax, and start incorporating mindfulness into your workday today.

Chapter 3: Implementing Mindfulness Techniques

Breathing Exercises for Stress Relief

In today's fast-paced work environments, stress is a common experience for many employees. The demands of deadlines, meetings, and high expectations can often leave individuals feeling overwhelmed and anxious. However, there are simple and effective ways to manage workplace stress, and one powerful tool is through the practice of breathing exercises. By incorporating breathing exercises into your daily routine, you can reduce stress levels, improve focus, and increase overall well-being.

Breathing exercises are a valuable tool for stress relief because they help activate the body's relaxation response. When we are stressed, our bodies go into a fight-or-flight mode, which can increase heart rate, blood pressure, and muscle tension. By practicing deep breathing exercises, we can stimulate the parasympathetic nervous system, also known as the rest-and-digest response, which helps calm the body and mind. This can lead to decreased levels of stress hormones and an overall sense of relaxation.

One simple breathing exercise that can be practiced in the workplace is diaphragmatic breathing. To practice this technique, sit or stand in a comfortable position and place one hand on your abdomen. Inhale deeply through your nose, allowing your abdomen to expand as you breathe in. Exhale slowly through your mouth, feeling your abdomen contract. Repeat this process for several breaths, focusing on the rise and fall of your abdomen. This exercise can help regulate your breathing, reduce stress, and increase oxygen flow to the brain.

Another effective breathing exercise for stress relief is the 4-7-8 technique. This involves inhaling for a count of 4, holding your breath for a count of 7, and exhaling for a count of 8. This exercise can help slow down your breathing, calm your mind, and promote relaxation. By incorporating this technique into your daily routine, you can build resilience to stress and improve your ability to cope with challenging situations in the workplace.

Incorporating breathing exercises into your daily routine can have a profound impact on your overall well-being and productivity in the workplace. By taking a few minutes each day to practice deep breathing techniques, you can reduce stress levels, increase focus, and improve your ability to handle challenging situations. So the next time you're feeling overwhelmed at work, take a moment to pause, breathe deeply, and allow yourself to relax and succeed.

Body Scan Meditation for Relaxation

Body scan meditation is a powerful technique that can help individuals in the workplace manage stress and improve overall well-being. This practice involves focusing on each part of the body, starting from the top of the head and moving down to the toes, in order to bring awareness and relaxation to each area. By tuning in to the physical sensations in the body, individuals can release tension and promote a sense of calm and relaxation.

To begin a body scan meditation, find a quiet and comfortable space where you can sit or lie down without any distractions. Close your eyes and take a few deep breaths to center yourself. Start by bringing your attention to the top of your head and slowly move down, noticing any areas of tension or discomfort along the way. As you scan each part of your body, take note of any sensations you may be feeling without judgment.

As you continue the body scan, be sure to breathe deeply and slowly, allowing yourself to fully relax and let go of any stress or tension you may be holding onto. Focus on each body part individually, bringing awareness and attention to the sensations present in that area. By doing so, you can release physical and mental tension, allowing yourself to enter a state of deep relaxation and peace.

Body scan meditation is a valuable tool for managing workplace stress, as it helps individuals to tune into their bodies and release tension that may be contributing to their stress levels. By practicing this technique regularly, individuals can learn to recognize when their body is holding onto stress and take steps to release it before it becomes overwhelming. This can lead to improved focus, productivity, and overall well-being in the workplace.

In conclusion, body scan meditation is a simple yet effective practice that can help individuals in the workplace manage stress and promote relaxation. By bringing awareness to each part of the body and releasing tension, individuals can experience a sense of calm and peace that can carry over into their workday. Incorporating body scan meditation into your daily routine can be a powerful tool for managing workplace stress and improving overall mental and physical well-being.

Mindful Walking for Mental Clarity

Mindful walking is a powerful practice that can help you achieve mental clarity and reduce workplace stress. By focusing on each step, breath, and sensation as you walk, you can bring your attention fully to the present moment, allowing your mind to let go of worries and distractions. This simple yet effective technique can help you recenter and refocus, providing a much-needed break from the demands of the workplace.

To practice mindful walking for mental clarity, start by finding a quiet and peaceful place to walk. This could be a park, a garden, or even just a quiet hallway in your office building. As you begin walking, pay attention to each step you take. Notice the sensation of your feet making contact with the ground, the movement of your muscles, and the rhythm of your breath. By bringing your full attention to these sensations, you can quiet the chatter of your mind and find a sense of calm and clarity.

As you continue walking mindfully, you may begin to notice the thoughts and emotions that arise in your mind. Instead of getting caught up in these thoughts, simply acknowledge them and let them pass by, returning your focus to the present moment. This practice of non-judgmental awareness can help you cultivate a sense of inner peace and clarity, allowing you to navigate the challenges of the workplace with greater ease.

Mindful walking can be especially helpful during times of stress or overwhelm at work. By taking a few minutes to step away and practice this simple technique, you can reset your mind and body, allowing yourself to approach your work with a renewed sense of focus and energy. With regular practice, you may find that mindful walking becomes a valuable tool in managing workplace stress and promoting mental well-being.

Incorporating mindful walking into your daily routine can have lasting benefits for your mental clarity and overall well-being. By taking the time to slow down, connect with your body, and bring your attention fully to the present moment, you can create a sense of calm and balance that will serve you well in the workplace and beyond. So next time you feel overwhelmed or stressed at work, consider taking a mindful walk to clear your mind and find a sense of mental clarity.

Chapter 4: Creating a Mindful Work Environment

Encouraging Mindfulness Practices in the Workplace

In today's fast-paced work environment, workplace stress is a common issue that many employees face on a daily basis. The constant pressure to meet deadlines, handle difficult clients, and juggle multiple tasks can take a toll on one's mental and physical well-being. However, incorporating mindfulness practices into the workplace can help employees manage stress, improve focus, and foster a more positive work environment.

Encouraging mindfulness practices in the workplace involves creating a supportive and inclusive culture that values the well-being of employees. Employers can start by offering mindfulness training sessions or workshops to introduce employees to the concept and benefits of mindfulness. These sessions can teach employees techniques such as deep breathing, meditation, and body scans that can help them relax, reduce stress, and improve their overall well-being.

Another way to encourage mindfulness practices in the workplace is to create designated spaces for employees to practice mindfulness. This could include setting up a quiet room or meditation area where employees can go to relax and recharge during the workday. Providing resources such as guided meditation apps or mindfulness coloring books can also help employees incorporate mindfulness into their daily routines.

In addition to providing resources and training, employers can lead by example and incorporate mindfulness practices into their own daily routines. By demonstrating the benefits of mindfulness, employers can inspire their employees to follow suit and make mindfulness a regular part of their workday. This can help create a more positive and supportive work environment where employees feel valued and supported in managing their stress.

Overall, encouraging mindfulness practices in the workplace can benefit both employees and employers by reducing workplace stress, improving focus and productivity, and fostering a more positive work environment. By creating a culture that values mindfulness and well-being, employers can help their employees thrive in today's fast-paced work environment.

Mindful Communication Techniques

In today's fast-paced and high-pressure work environments, effective communication is key to managing workplace stress. Mindful communication techniques can help individuals navigate difficult conversations, foster positive relationships, and reduce stress levels. By incorporating mindfulness into our daily interactions, we can improve our communication skills and create a more harmonious work environment.

One of the fundamental principles of mindful communication is active listening. This involves fully engaging with the speaker, paying attention to their words, tone, and body language. By practicing active listening, we can better understand the perspectives of others, build trust, and avoid misunderstandings. This can help prevent conflicts and reduce stress in the workplace.

Another important aspect of mindful communication is being present in the moment. This means focusing on the conversation at hand and avoiding distractions such as checking emails or thinking about other tasks. By being fully present, we can give our full attention to the speaker and respond thoughtfully, rather than reacting impulsively. This can lead to more meaningful and productive conversations, ultimately reducing stress levels for all parties involved.

Mindful communication also involves being aware of our own emotions and reactions. By taking a moment to pause and reflect before responding, we can choose our words more carefully and communicate more effectively. This can help prevent misunderstandings and conflicts, as well as reduce stress by promoting a sense of calm and control in challenging situations.

Overall, incorporating mindful communication techniques into our daily interactions can help us manage workplace stress more effectively. By practicing active listening, being present in the moment, and being aware of our emotions, we can improve our communication skills, build stronger relationships, and create a more positive work environment. By taking the time to cultivate mindful communication habits, we can reduce stress and enhance our overall well-being in the workplace.

Mindful Eating for Stress Management

Mindful eating is a powerful tool for managing stress in the workplace. When we are stressed, we often turn to food for comfort or distraction. However, this can lead to mindless eating, where we consume food without being fully present in the moment. By practicing mindful eating, we can cultivate a greater awareness of our eating habits and make more conscious choices about what and how much we eat.

One of the key principles of mindful eating is paying attention to the sensations of eating, such as the taste, texture, and smell of the food. By focusing on these sensory experiences, we can fully savor our food and derive greater enjoyment from it. This can help to reduce stress by allowing us to slow down and appreciate the present moment, rather than rushing through our meals in a state of distraction.

Another important aspect of mindful eating is tuning into our body's hunger and fullness cues. Often, we eat out of habit or in response to emotional triggers, rather than true physical hunger. By listening to our body and eating only when we are hungry, we can avoid overeating and feeling sluggish or guilty afterwards. This can help to reduce stress by fostering a healthier relationship with food and our bodies.

Mindful eating can also help us to break free from the cycle of emotional eating, where we use food as a coping mechanism for stress or negative emotions. By becoming more aware of our eating habits and the emotions that drive them, we can begin to make more conscious choices about how we nourish ourselves. This can lead to a greater sense of control and empowerment in managing stress, as we learn to respond to our emotions in more constructive ways.

In conclusion, mindful eating is a valuable tool for managing stress in the workplace. By cultivating a greater awareness of our eating habits, tuning into our body's hunger and fullness cues, and breaking free from emotional eating patterns, we can develop a healthier relationship with food and reduce stress in our daily lives. Incorporating mindfulness into our eating habits can help us to savor our food, make more conscious choices, and ultimately feel more balanced and in control of our well-being.

Chapter 5: Overcoming Challenges and Maintaining Mindfulness

Dealing with Resistance to Mindfulness

Dealing with resistance to mindfulness can be a common challenge in the workplace, especially when it comes to managing stress. Many employees may initially be hesitant to embrace mindfulness practices, viewing them as a waste of time or not applicable to their busy work schedules. However, it is important for employers and employees alike to recognize the benefits of mindfulness in reducing workplace stress and improving overall well-being.

One way to address resistance to mindfulness in the workplace is to provide education and training on the benefits of mindfulness. By offering workshops or seminars that explain the science behind mindfulness and its impact on stress management, employees may be more inclined to give it a try. It is important to emphasize that mindfulness is not a one-size-fits-all solution, but rather a tool that can be customized to fit individual needs and preferences.

Another strategy for dealing with resistance to mindfulness is to lead by example. Employers and managers can demonstrate their commitment to mindfulness by incorporating it into their own daily routines and encouraging others to do the same. By showing that mindfulness is valued and supported within the organization, employees may feel more comfortable exploring mindfulness practices themselves.

It is also important to create a supportive environment for mindfulness in the workplace. This can include setting aside dedicated time and space for mindfulness activities, such as meditation or yoga classes, and encouraging open communication about the benefits of mindfulness. By fostering a culture of mindfulness, employees may feel more motivated to overcome their resistance and give it a try.

In conclusion, dealing with resistance to mindfulness in the workplace requires a combination of education, leadership, and support. By providing resources and encouragement for mindfulness practices, employers can help employees better manage workplace stress and improve their overall well-being. Ultimately, embracing mindfulness can lead to a more productive and positive work environment for everyone involved.

Strategies for Making Mindfulness a Habit

In order to effectively manage workplace stress with mindfulness, it's important to develop strategies that help incorporate mindfulness into your daily routine. Making mindfulness a habit can have a significant impact on reducing stress levels and improving overall well-being. Here are some strategies to help you make mindfulness a habit in the workplace.

First and foremost, set aside dedicated time each day for mindfulness practice. Whether it's first thing in the morning, during your lunch break, or before bed, carving out time for mindfulness can help you stay consistent and make it a regular part of your routine. By prioritizing mindfulness practice in your schedule, you can ensure that it becomes a habit rather than something you do sporadically.

Another strategy for making mindfulness a habit is to incorporate it into your daily activities. This can include practicing mindfulness while walking to meetings, taking deep breaths before responding to emails, or simply taking a moment to pause and reset throughout the day. By weaving mindfulness into your daily tasks, you can reinforce the habit and make it a natural part of your workday.

Creating visual reminders can also help reinforce mindfulness as a habit in the workplace. This could be as simple as placing a sticky note on your computer screen with a mindfulness reminder, setting a mindfulness app as your screensaver, or keeping a small object on your desk that serves as a mindfulness cue. These visual reminders can help keep mindfulness top of mind and encourage you to practice it regularly.

Additionally, finding an accountability partner can be a helpful strategy for making mindfulness a habit. Whether it's a coworker, friend, or family member, having someone to check in with can provide motivation and support as you work to establish mindfulness as a habit. By sharing your mindfulness goals and progress with someone else, you can stay accountable and stay on track with your mindfulness practice.

Finally, be patient with yourself as you work to make mindfulness a habit in the workplace. Building a new habit takes time and consistency, so it's important to be gentle and compassionate with yourself throughout the process. Remember that mindfulness is a skill that can be developed over time, and with practice and dedication, you can make mindfulness a regular part of your workday and effectively manage workplace stress.

Coping with Setbacks and Maintaining a Mindful Outlook

In the fast-paced world of the workplace, setbacks are bound to happen. Whether it's something that didn't go as planned or a conflict with a colleague, navigating these challenges can be stressful. However, it's important to remember that setbacks are a natural part of any professional journey and can provide valuable learning experiences. By maintaining a mindful outlook, you can cope with setbacks in a healthy and productive way.

One of the key strategies for coping with setbacks is to practice mindfulness. Mindfulness involves being fully present in the moment and accepting things as they are, without judgment. When faced with a setback, take a moment to pause, breathe, and center yourself. This can help you to approach the situation with a calm and clear mind, rather than reacting impulsively out of frustration or anxiety.

Another important aspect of coping with setbacks is to maintain a positive attitude. It can be easy to fall into a negative mindset when things don't go as planned, but dwelling on the negative aspects of a situation will only make it harder to move forward. Instead, try to focus on the lessons that can be learned from the setback and look for opportunities for growth and improvement.

It's also helpful to seek support from others when dealing with setbacks. Talking to a trusted colleague or mentor can provide valuable perspective and advice on how to navigate the situation. Additionally, reaching out to a therapist or counselor can be beneficial for processing your emotions and developing coping strategies for managing workplace stress.

By practicing mindfulness, maintaining a positive attitude, and seeking support from others, you can cope with setbacks in a healthy and productive way. Remember that setbacks are a natural part of any professional journey, and by approaching them with a mindful outlook, you can learn and grow from these experiences. Stay resilient and keep moving forward, knowing that you have the tools to navigate any challenges that come your way in the workplace.

Chapter 6: Succeeding in the Workplace with Mindfulness

Improving Focus and Productivity through Mindfulness

In today's fast-paced work environment, it can be challenging to stay focused and productive amidst the constant demands and distractions. However, by incorporating mindfulness practices into your daily routine, you can improve your ability to concentrate and enhance your overall productivity. Mindfulness involves being fully present in the moment, without judgment, and can help reduce stress and anxiety while increasing mental clarity and focus.

One way to improve focus and productivity through mindfulness is to start your day with a brief meditation or breathing exercise. Taking just a few minutes to center yourself before diving into your work can help clear your mind and set a positive tone for the day ahead. By practicing mindfulness regularly, you can train your brain to better filter out distractions and stay more focused on the task at hand.

Another helpful mindfulness technique for improving focus and productivity is to practice mindful eating. Instead of mindlessly scarfing down your lunch at your desk, take the time to savor each bite, paying attention to the flavors, textures, and sensations in your mouth. By eating mindfully, you can reduce stress, improve digestion, and enhance your overall well-being, leading to increased focus and productivity throughout the day.

In addition to incorporating mindfulness practices into your daily routine, it's important to create a work environment that supports focus and productivity. This may involve cleaning your workspace, minimizing distractions, and setting boundaries with coworkers to limit interruptions. By creating a calm and organized work environment, you can help cultivate a sense of mindfulness and promote greater focus and productivity in your day-to-day tasks.

In conclusion, by incorporating mindfulness practices into your daily routine and creating a supportive work environment, you can improve your focus and productivity in the workplace. Mindfulness can help reduce stress, increase mental clarity, and enhance overall well-being, leading to a more positive and productive work experience. By taking the time to practice mindfulness and cultivate a sense of presence in your daily activities, you can better manage workplace stress and achieve greater success in your professional endeavors.

Enhancing Creativity and Problem-Solving Skills

In today's fast-paced work environment, it is essential for employees to possess strong creativity and problem-solving skills to navigate through the challenges they face daily. Enhancing these skills not only benefits individuals in their professional growth but also contributes to the overall success of the organization. We will explore strategies and techniques to help you cultivate your creativity and hone your problem-solving abilities, ultimately leading to a more productive and fulfilling work experience.

One way to enhance creativity and problem-solving skills is to practice mindfulness. Mindfulness involves paying attention to the present moment without judgment, allowing you to fully engage with your thoughts and feelings. By practicing mindfulness, you can tap into your creative potential and approach problem-solving tasks with a clear and focused mind.

Another effective way to enhance creativity and problem-solving skills is to engage in activities that stimulate your mind and spark your imagination. This could include brainstorming sessions with colleagues, taking on new projects or tasks that push you out of your comfort zone, or participating in creative workshops or training programs. By exposing yourself to new experiences and ideas, you can expand your thinking and develop innovative solutions to complex problems.

Collaboration is key when it comes to enhancing creativity and problem-solving skills in the workplace. By working with others, you can leverage different perspectives and expertise to generate new ideas and approaches to solving problems. Collaborative problem-solving not only fosters a sense of teamwork and camaraderie among colleagues but also leads to more effective and efficient solutions that benefit the organization as a whole.

In conclusion, enhancing creativity and problem-solving skills is crucial for managing workplace stress and achieving success in today's competitive work environment. By practicing mindfulness, engaging in stimulating activities, and collaborating with others, you can unlock your creative potential and develop effective strategies for overcoming challenges at work. By cultivating these skills, you will not only improve your own job performance but also contribute to a more innovative and productive workplace culture.

Building Resilience and Managing Workplace Stress Effectively

In today's work environment, it is essential to build resilience and manage workplace stress effectively. Stress in the workplace can have detrimental effects on both physical and mental health, leading to decreased productivity and overall job satisfaction. By implementing mindfulness techniques, individuals can learn to navigate stressors with grace and composure, ultimately improving their performance and well-being in the workplace.

One key aspect of building resilience in the workplace is developing a mindfulness practice. Mindfulness involves being present in the moment, without judgment or attachment to thoughts or emotions. By practicing mindfulness regularly, individuals can learn to respond to stressors in a more calm and composed manner, rather than reacting impulsively. This can lead to improved communication, problem-solving skills, and overall job satisfaction.

Another important aspect of managing workplace stress effectively is setting boundaries and practicing self-care. It is crucial for individuals to prioritize their mental and physical well-being in order to perform at their best in the workplace. This may involve setting limits on work hours, taking breaks throughout the day, and engaging in activities that promote relaxation and stress relief. By taking care of themselves, individuals can better manage stress and build resilience in the face of challenges.

Furthermore, building a strong support network in the workplace can also help individuals manage stress effectively. By fostering positive relationships with colleagues and supervisors, individuals can feel more supported and connected in their work environment. This support system can provide a valuable source of encouragement and guidance during difficult times, helping individuals navigate stressors with greater ease.

Overall, by incorporating mindfulness practices, setting boundaries, practicing self-care, and building a support network, individuals can effectively manage workplace stress and build resilience in the face of challenges. By taking proactive steps to prioritize their well-being, individuals can thrive in the workplace and achieve success in their professional endeavors.

Chapter 7: Mindfulness Resources for Continued Growth

Books and Online Resources for Mindfulness

In today's demanding work environments, it is crucial for employees to find effective ways to manage stress and maintain a sense of balance and mindfulness. One valuable resource for achieving this is books and online resources that focus on mindfulness practices. These resources provide practical tips, techniques, and strategies for cultivating mindfulness in the workplace, ultimately helping individuals to better cope with stress and improve their overall well-being.

Books on mindfulness can be a significant source of inspiration and guidance for individuals looking to incorporate mindfulness into their daily lives. These books often provide in-depth explanations of mindfulness principles, as well as practical exercises and meditations that can help individuals develop their mindfulness skills. Some well-known books on mindfulness include "The Miracle of Mindfulness" by Thich Nhat Hanh, "Wherever You Go, There You Are" by Jon Kabat-Zinn, and "The Power of Now" by Eckhart Tolle.

Online resources for mindfulness offer a wealth of information and tools that can be accessed conveniently from anywhere with an internet connection. Websites, podcasts, and online courses dedicated to mindfulness provide a variety of resources, including guided meditations, mindfulness exercises, and articles on stress management and well-being. Some popular online resources for mindfulness include Mindful.org, Headspace, and Calm.

By utilizing books and online resources for mindfulness, employees can gain valuable insights and practical tools for managing workplace stress more effectively. These resources can help individuals develop greater self-awareness, emotional regulation, and resilience in the face of workplace challenges. By incorporating mindfulness practices into their daily routines, employees can experience reduced stress levels, improved focus and productivity, and enhanced overall well-being.

In conclusion, books and online resources for mindfulness offer valuable support and guidance for individuals seeking to manage workplace stress and cultivate mindfulness in their daily lives. By exploring these resources and incorporating mindfulness practices into their routines, employees can develop the skills and strategies needed to navigate the demands of the modern workplace with greater ease and resilience. Embracing mindfulness in the workplace can lead to a more balanced, productive, and fulfilling work experience for employees across all industries.

Mindfulness Workshops and Retreats

Mindfulness workshops and retreats offer a valuable opportunity for employees to learn how to effectively manage workplace stress. These programs typically focus on teaching participants how to cultivate mindfulness, which is the practice of paying attention to the present moment without judgment. By incorporating mindfulness into their daily routines, employees can reduce stress and improve their overall well-being.

Workshops often include a variety of activities such as guided meditation, yoga, and breathing exercises. These practices help employees develop greater self-awareness and emotional regulation, allowing them to respond to stressful situations in a more calm and composed manner. By learning how to stay present and focused, employees can avoid becoming overwhelmed by the demands of their work environment.

Retreats provide employees with a more immersive experience, allowing them to disconnect from their daily routines and fully immerse themselves in mindfulness practices. This extended period of time away from the office can be incredibly rejuvenating, allowing participants to recharge and return to work with a renewed sense of focus and clarity. Retreats often include group discussions, nature walks, and mindfulness exercises, all designed to help employees deepen their mindfulness practice and develop new coping strategies for managing stress.

Both workshops and retreats offer employees a supportive and non-judgmental environment in which to explore mindfulness and its benefits. Participants are encouraged to share their experiences and insights with one another, fostering a sense of community and connection. This shared journey of self-discovery can be incredibly empowering, helping employees to realize that they are not alone in their struggles with workplace stress.

Overall, mindfulness workshops and retreats can be a powerful tool for helping employees manage workplace stress. By learning how to cultivate mindfulness and practice self-care techniques, employees can create a more balanced and fulfilling work life. These programs provide a safe space for employees to explore new ways of coping with stress and build resilience in the face of workplace challenges.

Finding Support and Accountability in Your Mindfulness Practice

In the fast-paced world of the workplace, managing stress can often feel like an uphill battle. However, finding support and accountability in your mindfulness practice can be a game-changer when it comes to reducing workplace stress. By creating a supportive network of colleagues or friends who are also practicing mindfulness, you can hold each other accountable and stay motivated to prioritize self-care even during the busiest of workdays.

One way to find support in your mindfulness practice is to join a workplace mindfulness group or create one yourself. This can be as simple as setting up a weekly lunchtime meditation session or organizing a book club to discuss mindfulness techniques and strategies. By coming together with like-minded individuals, you can share experiences, offer encouragement, and hold each other accountable for sticking to your mindfulness goals.

Another effective way to find support in your mindfulness practice is to enlist the help of a mindfulness coach or mentor. These individuals can provide guidance, support, and accountability as you navigate the challenges of incorporating mindfulness into your daily routine. Whether through one-on-one sessions or group workshops, a mindfulness coach can help you stay on track and make meaningful progress in your mindfulness practice.

In addition to finding support in your mindfulness practice, accountability is also crucial for managing workplace stress effectively. By setting specific goals and deadlines for your mindfulness practice, you can hold yourself accountable for making self-care a priority. Whether it's committing to meditating for 10 minutes each morning or taking a mindful walk during your lunch break, accountability can help you stay focused and motivated to reduce stress in the workplace.

In conclusion, finding support and accountability in your mindfulness practice is essential for managing workplace stress. By creating a supportive network, joining a mindfulness group, enlisting the help of a coach, and setting specific goals, you can stay motivated and on track to prioritize self-care even in the most stressful work environments. With the right support and accountability, you can cultivate a mindfulness practice that helps you thrive in the workplace and beyond.

Chapter 8: Conclusion

Recap of Key Points

We will recap some of the key points discussed throughout the book "Breathe, Relax, Succeed: Managing Workplace Stress with Mindfulness" that are essential for managing workplace stress effectively. By implementing these strategies, you can create a more balanced and harmonious work environment for yourself and your colleagues.

First and foremost, it is crucial to recognize the signs of workplace stress and understand how it impacts your mental and physical well-being. By being mindful of your stress triggers, you can take proactive steps to address them before they escalate. Remember to listen to your body and emotions, as they often provide valuable insights into your stress levels.

Secondly, practicing mindfulness techniques such as deep breathing, meditation, and yoga can help you stay grounded and present in the moment. These practices can help you manage your stress response and cultivate a sense of calm and clarity amidst chaos. By incorporating mindfulness into your daily routine, you can build resilience and cope more effectively with workplace challenges.

Additionally, setting boundaries and prioritizing self-care are essential for maintaining a healthy work-life balance. Learn to say no to tasks that overwhelm you and make time for activities that nourish your mind, body, and soul. Taking breaks throughout the day and getting regular exercise can also help reduce stress and boost your overall well-being.

Furthermore, fostering positive relationships with your coworkers and seeking support when needed can make a significant difference in how you navigate workplace stress. Remember that you are not alone in experiencing stress, and reaching out for help is a sign of strength, not weakness. By building a supportive network and practicing empathy and compassion, you can create a more collaborative and harmonious work environment.

In conclusion, managing workplace stress with mindfulness requires a holistic approach that encompasses self-awareness, self-care, and social support. By incorporating the key points discussed in this book into your daily routine, you can cultivate a sense of balance, resilience, and well-being in the workplace. Remember that you have the power to transform your relationship with stress and create a more fulfilling and sustainable work experience for yourself and those around you.

Final Thoughts on Managing Workplace Stress with Mindfulness

In conclusion, managing workplace stress with mindfulness is a powerful tool that can help individuals navigate the challenges of the modern work environment. By incorporating mindfulness practices into our daily routines, we can cultivate a greater sense of calm, clarity, and resilience in the face of stressors. It is important to remember that mindfulness is not a quick fix or a one-size-fits-all solution, but rather a skill that requires practice and dedication to see lasting results.

One of the key takeaways from this book is the importance of self-awareness in managing workplace stress. By tuning into our thoughts, emotions, and physical sensations, we can begin to recognize the early warning signs of stress and take proactive steps to address them before they escalate. Mindfulness can help us develop a greater sense of self-awareness and emotional intelligence, allowing us to respond to stress in a more adaptive and effective manner.

Another important aspect of managing workplace stress with mindfulness is the cultivation of a non-judgmental attitude towards ourselves and others. By approaching stress with compassion, curiosity, and acceptance, we can create a more supportive and nurturing work environment that encourages growth and resilience. Mindfulness teaches us to let go of perfectionism and self-criticism, and instead focus on progress, learning, and personal growth.

It is also worth noting that managing workplace stress with mindfulness is not a solo endeavor. By fostering a culture of mindfulness in the workplace, organizations can support their employees in developing the skills and resources needed to cope with stress and thrive in their roles. Leaders can set the tone by modeling mindfulness practices and creating opportunities for employees to engage in mindfulness training, workshops, and group activities.

Ultimately, managing workplace stress with mindfulness is a journey of self-discovery and personal growth that can lead to greater well-being, productivity, and job satisfaction. By incorporating mindfulness practices into our daily lives, we can cultivate a greater sense of balance, resilience, and fulfillment in the workplace. I hope that the insights and strategies shared in this book will inspire you to embark on your own mindfulness journey and experience the transformative power of mindfulness in managing workplace stress.

Vivamus vestibulum ntulla nec ante.

Lorem ipsum dolor sit amet, consectetur adipiscing elit, sed do eiusmod tempor incididunt ut labore et dolore magna aliqua. Ut enim ad minim veniam, quis nostrud exercitationullamco laboris nisi ut aliquip ex ea commodo consequat. Duis aute irure dolor in reprehenderit involuptate velit esse cillum dolore eu fugiat nulla pariatur. Excepteur sint occaecat cupidatat nonproident, sunt in culpa qui officia deserunt mollit anim id est laborum.

Sed egestas, ante et vulputate volutpat, eros pede semper est, vitae luctus metus libero eu augue. Morbi purus libero, faucibus adipiscing, commodo quis, gravida id, est. Sed lectus. Praesent elementum hendrerit tortor. Sed semper lorem at felis. Vestibulum volutpat, lacus a ultrices sagittis, mi neque euismod dui, eu pulvinar nunc sapien ornare nisl. Phasellus pede arcu, dapibus eu, fermentum et, dapibus sed, urna.